THE SIMPLE DOCTOR SERIES

I0086352

Take a
Simple Drive
to a
Healthier Life

and Live Longer Too!

DR. ROGER SMITH

Copyright © 2017 Roger Smith
Revised 2020

Cover image: copyright: profile_inspirestock, 123RF Stock Photo
Typeset & Edited by Power of Words

ISBN-13: 978-0-6480930-0-8 (paperback)

Cataloguing-in-Publication data:

Creator: Smith, Roger, 1960- author.
Title: Take a simple drive to a healthier life : and live longer too! /
Dr. Roger Smith.

Subjects: Health.
Well-being.
Longevity.

Book website: **thesimpledoctor.info**
Printed in Australia
Please give feedback on the book
at your favourite book merchant.

Dr Roger Smith is to be commended for writing a book whose theme was driven by an encounter with a patient who seemed to value his car more than his heart.

The message is quite simple....look after yourself, try to understand the role of environmental and behavioural factors in the causation of disease, factors over which you the patient has control. Undertake regular check-ups and take control of your health through diet, exercise, avoidance of smoking, alcohol etc. and early identification of problems before they become unmanageable. The book is written in an engaging style for the layman and is very reader friendly.

PROFESSOR LEON PITERMAN AM
Professor of General Practice
Director, China Programs
Monash Institute for Health & Clinical Education (MIHCE)

To my original partners in general practice, from 1990 – Sam, Guenter and Tom – who showed me that medicine can be both serious and fun.

Illustrations

Table of Contents

Preface

❦

Working in general practice for over twenty-five years has taught me a great deal. Most things are routine and yet you have to have your wits about you. The next seemingly uncomplicated patient may end up being anything but simple.

It was a Sunday about midday. Our practice had always been open long hours and this guaranteed you would always see a variety of interesting patients. I called the next patient — Nic, a man in his mid seventies — into the room. He sat down and began to tell me about some chest pain he was experiencing. It had started around midnight, about 12 hours earlier, while he had been watching football.

Chest pain in anyone over forty may have a serious cause. As he continued his story of chest pain it became clear that this may well be heart related. An examination revealed nothing of note. An ECG (heart tracing) was then performed. Sure enough, this confirmed my suspicions — yes — he was having a heart attack and would have to go to hospital via ambulance NOW.

When I advised him of this, he was surprised, shocked and very upset. I tried to reassure him but he insisted that he would have to go home first. When I asked him why, it was all about his car! He simply could not cope with the idea of leaving it in the clinic car park.

So that was it — he was more concerned about his car than his heart! Can you believe it? Sensing how big a deal this was for him, and knowing how important it is to keep a patient calm, I told him not to worry. I would drive his car home at the end of the day and then simply give the keys to his neighbour. Once I offered to do this, he seemed to relax, well as best he could in the circumstances given the life-threatening cardiac event.

The paramedics arrived, assessed his condition and he happily went off in the ambulance — comfortable knowing that his beloved car would be well looked after!

I thought that this was simplest way out of the problem as his house was only five minutes' drive away. All I had to do now was to work until nine pm, then take his car home — what could possibly go wrong?

When I had completed the day's work, I organised for my receptionist Janet to simply follow me to Nic's house in her car. By the time we left the building it was dark. I started the car and as I began to drive out of the parking lot I noticed that something was wrong. The car was veering a little to the left and it took a great effort to keep the car straight. It was no better on the road and as I turned the first corner I realised what the problem might be. 'Don't tell me it's a flat tyre,' I thought to myself.

I pulled to a halt near a street light to check, while Janet in her car behind wondered why I had stopped and turned my hazard lights on. Yep, sure enough, a flat tyre — flat as a pancake!

Something that should have been so easy had suddenly become a little bit more complicated. I asked Janet to shine her car lights to help illuminate the scene. Now, to change a tyre! I had not done this for many years but luckily changing a tyre is like riding a bike — once mastered — never forgotten. I just hoped that everything was where it should be and that the spare was inflated.

I should not have worried as Nic was obviously very methodical about all aspects of his car. Before long, we were back on the road and the procession of two cars made its way to Nic's house. There the car was safely parked in his driveway and the keys handed over to the amused neighbour. He had never seen such grand service.

I later rang the hospital to enquire about Nic's condition. I was advised that he had indeed suffered a heart attack, but more importantly, that he was in a stable condition. I was able to reassure him via the nursing staff that his beloved car was safe and tucked in at home after its own health scare.

So this whole funny saga made me ponder. Why indeed do some

people look after their cars much better than they care for themselves?

Imagine how well you might look after your car if it had to serve you for decades? Not for just five or ten years, but for twenty years or more! New and purring easily at first, much care and attention would be needed to make it last for the long haul. Remember, all classic cars were once new and shiny... but most of their contemporaries end up on the scrap-heap due to neglect or simply rusting out in the end.

Why do people often neglect their own bodies — their very own personal vehicle, which by its nature has to be with them for their whole life? It is foolhardy in the extreme. The ultimate penalty of early death or avoidable premature disability may be the result.

The state of your own personal health has many contributing factors. Luck — including genetics — plays a large role. If the car you purchase comes from a renowned manufacturer, then chances are it will be a reliable car. Likewise, if there is a history of longevity in your family, that is great news for you.

Of course you can always buy a lemon, even from a good manufacturer. You could receive the equivalent misfortune in life and be struck down by some rare life-threatening illness or disability. Sadly, for some, grave misfortune is an overwhelming factor.

So, if the luck element can be appreciated and then removed from the equation, perhaps consider the following scenario. If you want your lifelong personal vehicle (your body) to last the journey, what should be your approach? How might you treat your body so that you do increase the chance of being a 'classic' in your later years?

Cars come with a user manual, but our bodies do not. We are taught some aspects of self-care by our parents and pick up other bits along the way. The result is not always a complete and accurate manual to go by. Hopefully the following discussion will at least fill some of the possible gaps in your own individual manual of knowledge.

Overloading

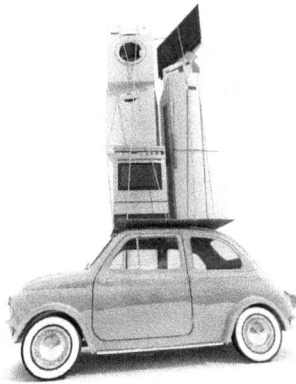

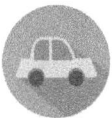

"Overloading can affect handling and stability and cause a crash in which you could be hurt or killed – follow all loading guidelines in this manual".

Fuel consumption is higher and there is more wear and tear on the car's brakes, tyres and suspension. A logical description that you will find in all car manuals. It makes a lot of sense.

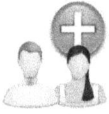 Overloading your body may also have dangerous repercussions — perhaps not immediately but almost certainly in the long run. The risk of developing many chronic health conditions is increased dramatically as the amount of body fat increases.

According to the Victorian Government's *Better Health Channel*, this is just a brief outline of some of the potential problems:

- high blood pressure
- atherosclerosis – fat lining the arteries
- cardiovascular disease – strokes and heart attacks
- some cancers including breast, endometrial and colon cancer
- type 2 diabetes
- gall bladder disease
- polycystic ovarian syndrome
- musculoskeletal problems, such as osteoarthritis and back pain
- stress incontinence
- sleep apnoea.

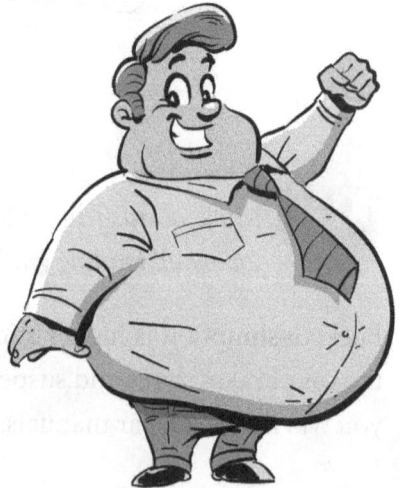

A Community Survey

To gauge how significant this problem was in my community, I performed a small study of my patients at the clinic. This informal study of one hundred consecutive patients over the age of 18 revealed the following:

24% were in the **normal weight** range

39% were **overweight**

37% were **obese**

None were classified as being underweight!

WEIGHT SURVEY - 100 PATIENTS

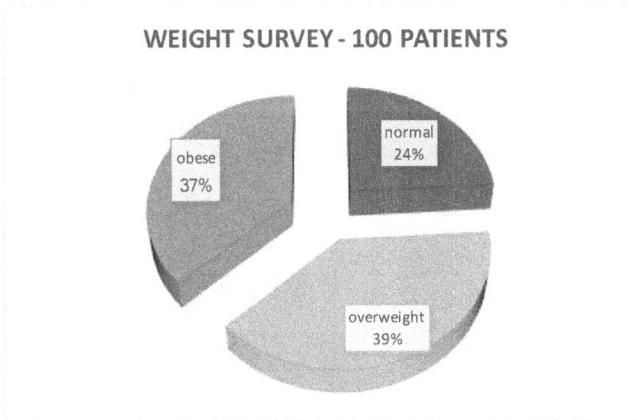

Put simply, less than one-third were in the normal weight range, which is astounding. By all reports, this normal sector may further reduce in the coming decades in most western countries.

These classifications (normal/overweight/obese) are quite broad but are still very useful. They are based on the concept of BMI — body mass index. This is a ratio of weight in kilograms divided by height in metres, squared.

This measure, although not perfect, at least gives you a guide as to where you are in regard to weight. Those who are very muscular may have high BMI, which does not have the same adverse problems associated with it.

Similarly, for children, there are charts available which help advise normal weight ranges for a given height and age.

HOW TO WORK OUT BMI

Less than 18.5	underweight
18.5 - 24.9	normal weight
25 - 29.9	overweight
30 +	obese
My current situation is: 83 kg 1.86 m	BMI: 83 divided by (1.86 x 1.86) = BMI 24

BMI: the ratio of weight (kg) divided by height (m) squared, i.e. BMI = kg / (m x m).

☺

So, you can see from this small survey that the problem of excess weight is an enormous issue.

I have, over the last decade or so, made a point to weigh the vast majority of my patients on a regular basis. There is often an initial humorous reluctance as some empty all their pockets before standing on my old green scales. Most patients do appreciate your taking the time to do this after you have discussed their primary reason for attending. By showing this concern, it encourages them to discuss this very important issue. In fact, more often than not, their weight may be a much more important factor in their long term health than their initial presenting problem of a sore throat or a nagging cough!

Once the weight and height is recorded, it provides a talking point. BMI can be calculated so quickly. If done for the first time, then at least some comment may be made about the current situation. If previous measures from past visits exist, then a graph on my computer screen will show any trend while providing an easy-to-understand picture.

I am quick to congratulate those whose weight is within the ideal or whose weight, although still highish, is trending downward.

Records dating back, say, fifteen years dramatically show the gradual effect of gaining a single kilogram per year... and it is not pretty!

When appropriate, the BMI result will then lead to a discussion about weight and how this can be managed. For at least the last ten years, I have used my own simple advice sheet to aid in the discussion (see later). This focuses on the three main issues: food intake / exercise / metabolism.

A Good Diet?

There are often excuses given as to why a good diet is not followed, or claims that it is being followed. We doctors hear many excuses as to why time is never found to go for a walk. Often the seasons are blamed — 'winter makes me eat more' or 'it is too wet/cold to walk'. For some, summer holds some hope as more salads will then be eaten, with resultant loss of weight. The salads may well be eaten, but so are too many other things!

Simply asking patients what they have for breakfast is often very revealing. The contrast in answers can be rather amazing. To many people's credit, they reply with the answer of porridge, or perhaps wholemeal toast. Sadly, some answers have been rather extreme. Replies have included:

- Nothing at all until midday — a common response
- Three shortbread biscuits with a cup of tea (lady in her seventies)
- Peanut butter on toast followed by a can of coke, with two more cans later in the day (lady aged in her thirties).

Waist circumference is another measure that may be used in conjunction with BMI. This is an indirect measure of visceral fat, which is thought to be a risk factor for many chronic diseases as is a raised BMI. There are different ranges for men and women, with a slight reduction for those of Asian background.

WAIST MEASUREMENT

	IDEAL	INCREASED RISK	HIGHER RISK
MEN	less than 94 cm	94 – 102 cm	> 102 cm
WOMEN	less than 80 cm	80 – 88 cm	> 88 cm

For both BMI and waist measurement, there are many online calculators available to assist you. These help in both the calculation as well as interpretation of the result.

So, how to address this issue of overloading?

The Three Main Issues

Assuming you have no underlying serious health issues, your current weight is determined by three main factors:-

- calorie intake (food)
- exercise (energy expenditure)
- metabolic rate

A. Calorie Intake

As a society, we tend to eat too much food, and in particular excess high-energy foods. It would be okay if we burnt this up, but we simply do not expend enough in an average day to do this. The result is expanding waistlines, as these calories are stored as fat.

My Road Map to Reduce Overloading
A simple patient info sheet

Essential Points

- It takes effort and planning
- 75% of the result is related to what you eat
- The end benefit to your health is enormous
- You do NOT need to buy expensive food products
- You need self-control and motivation

Serious about change? Then do the following:

1. **Avoid** or RARELY have any of these: cakes / sweet biscuits / lollies / chocolate / pies / pastries / all soft drinks / fruit juice / sugar in all drinks

2. Have **smaller meals**, i.e. 10% smaller, easily fitting on the average dinner plate

3. **Snacks** in-between-meals should be fruit or a dry biscuit/crackers — nil else

4. **Reduce** the amount of margarine used on toast

5. Drink more **water** / less alcohol ++

6. Have a healthy **breakfast**

7. **Weigh** weekly and record it. There will be ups and downs — the trend is the key!

8. **Exercise!**

If you are serious about trying to make a significant change, then you must follow the "Road Map to Reduce Overloading" as much as possible.

B.   Exercise

You need to do more, if your health allows. Ideally walk for at least 30 minutes, 4–5 times per week. It can be made up of smaller walks over the day if you prefer. Any increase on what you have been doing will make a difference. If you become breathless easily, walk more slowly. You will improve your fitness with time. Any activity, however brief, is beneficial.

Keep yourself busy during the day. Avoid prolonged periods of sitting.

C.   Metabolic Rate

This determines how much energy is required for your body to simply survive. This does vary from person to person. It is increased by exercise and smoking and reduced if you try to starve. For some people, missing breakfast tends to set the metabolic rate lower and may actually contribute to weight problems. For many, a healthy cereal — which might include hot porridge with some fruit — is actually a great, quick way to start the day and contribute to weight loss, when combined with the above tips.

To continue the car theme, consider metabolic rate to be like your car idling in the driveway. Even though at rest, the engine is still using fuel. Similarly, even while sitting, your body is using energy to keep the heart and lungs going and the billions of cells in you alive. So anything that makes the body use up more 'fuel' will be ideal for controlling your weight.

This difference in metabolic rate among people may explain in part why, despite seeming to eat similar amounts, one person can put on weight while another remains weight neutral. This can be so frustrating for those in the wrong group. Genetics can be so unfair!

Summary

What you eat... and how much you eat... are the key factors.

Make appropriate decisions about which foods you buy at the supermarket — so that when you are at home you will be less likely to eat the wrong things. Simply avoid the biscuit, cake, soft drink and sweet aisles while shopping. The supermarket is full of healthy foods, when you start looking. Make sure your trolley contents are at least 95% healthy as you line up at the checkout!

Reasonable weight loss is within your reach. This could range from ½ to 1 kg every one to three months, depending on your new eating pattern, the amount of exercise you do and your underlying metabolic rate.

That said, it does take great EFFORT to achieve any meaningful result and PERSISTENCE to maintain any loss. It is not easy to change long term, established patterns of behaviour.

Inability to exercise does NOT prevent weight loss. Any increase in your usual activity level will be of benefit. Addressing your diet is the key.

Any sustained loss will be of immense benefit to your health.

Rebound weight gain can occur if you resume your previous poor habits.

Real Patient Experiences

I have handed this *Road Map to Reduce Overloading* to numerous patients over the years and often asked them to nominate a predicted weight loss goal for the next six months.

Several years ago, I saw a patient (Barry – his real name!) who had proudly predicted that he could lose 5 kg in the next six months. At the two month mark I wrote to him, simply to remind him of the challenge and to encourage him.

When I saw him at the six month mark, he stated that he:

- Had achieved his initial weight loss goal of 5 kg;
- Had done absolutely nothing until he had received my reminder letter two months into the challenge (see over);
- Was greatly appreciative of the concern that I had shown by taking the time to write.

Barry then continued his new-found zest for fitness. When last seen, he was looking great, weighing 92 kg, down from his

---

The Simple Doctor Medical Practice

1st November 2015

Dear Barry,

Just a friendly reminder re the challenge to get your weight below 100 kg by February 2016.

Hope all is going well!

Yours sincerely,

Dr Roger Smith

---

original 106 kg in just over 12 months. Refer to graph 1.

This just proves that you need to do the following:

- Set reasonable targets
- Have a plan
- Be motivated to change — hopefully the thought of living longer is enough!

Hang on for the long haul... there will be a tendency for your weight to head back to where it used to be. Be prepared and accepting of this — and do what you can to combat this by keeping on track as best you can — remembering that even a sustained

5-10% weight loss is great for your long term health.

It will be very interesting to see how Barry goes in the long run!

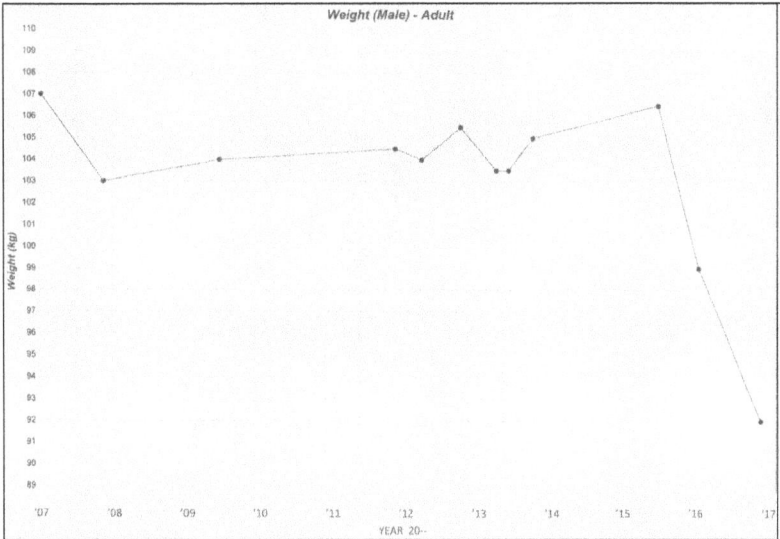

1. Barry — Target goal weight busted!

The fact is, while initial weight loss may seem easy for some, long term change and maintenance is a very hard task. Motivation and continued effort is crucial.

If you were to lose 10% of your previous weight, even if your new weight remains above the ideal range, a significant health benefit would still be achieved. Control of diabetes, lower blood pressure and lower cholesterol levels should be the result. For example, if you are 100 kg and the ideal range for your height is

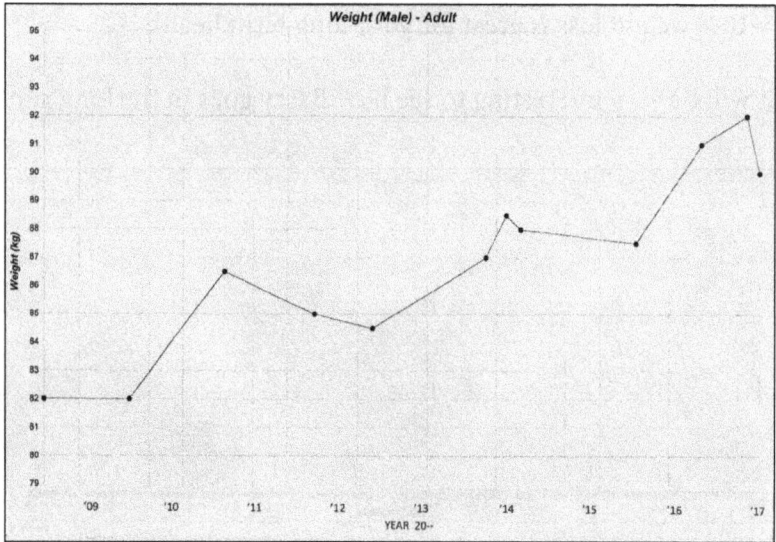

2. Graham — Procrastinated progress

65-80 kg, then reducing down to 90 kg AND staying there for the long haul is a tremendous result.

Far better than battling and getting down to 80 kg for six months, only then to relax and rebound back up to 100 kg or even more, as is what often happens.

It is not easy. Graham (not his real name) had been given the same advice as Barry and followed up with a reminder letter at the two-month mark. When seen next, there had been little change. He was quick to blame birthdays (everyone's, including his own), Christmas, and other external factors for his lack of success.

14

The drive for change must come from within. Yes, there are many factors that may make it a challenge, but real change does not come easy, nor is it easy to maintain it.

Interestingly, I saw Graham recently and he was keen to be weighed. Even though a little unmotivated at first, he had still lost a few kilograms, as seen in his weight graph (Graph no.2). Again, only time will tell what the end result will be.

Creeping Weight Gain

Graham's graph also reveals the effect of long term, slow weight gain. Sure, one kilogram weight gain by itself is nothing, but if you average one kilogram per year over eight years, the end result is not pretty. Let's hope he can maintain this new trend.

One last patient — Bob, who has done well. When he was in his mid-fifties, he had a major heart attack which left him with significant cardiac damage.

As a result, he became quite breathless on minimal exertion and had to cease work. He was advised by his heart specialist that he must lose weight and start to exercise if he wanted to extend his life for as long as possible.

Bob's graph (no.3) shows what he has been able to achieve by adhering to a new routine of healthy eating and daily walks. He's lost a total of 19 kg in 14 years!

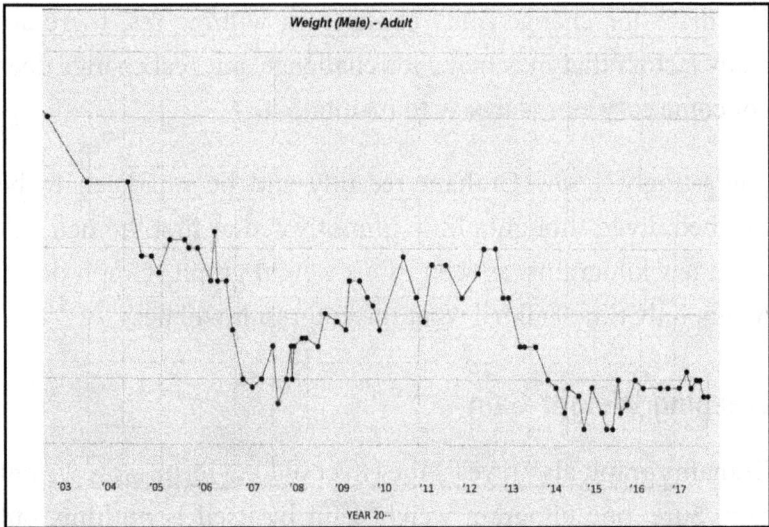

3. Bob — A new lighter, fitter man

He proudly steps on the scales every time he visits and is eager to see the result. Being lighter and fitter has enabled his life span to be extended.

2

Fuel

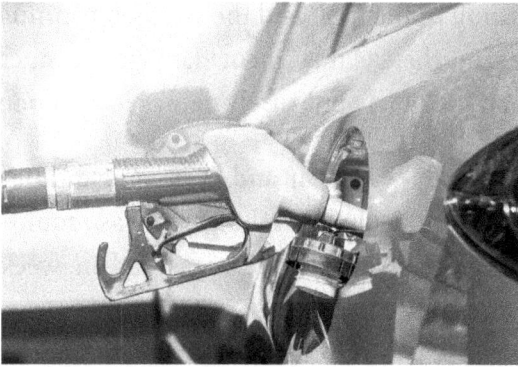

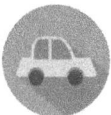

Every car has a recommended fuel that must be used — otherwise the engine will be severely damaged. Your vehicle may require unleaded fuel, LPG or diesel.

Recently a patient advised me that he had absentmindedly filled his diesel car with unleaded fuel. Luckily he realised this before he started the car. The end result was his beloved car had to be towed away and the fuel system drained to prevent any damage taking place.

Fuel

So, for a car this is easy... but *you* MUST use the correct fuel or there will be dire consequences.

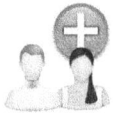

Fortunately, the body is very forgiving and is able to extract energy from most food sources. Really, unless you have ingested a clearly toxic substance, the body will be able to utilise it. It would be like having a car and putting almost anything in the tank and the car then running very well. In the long run, the car may incur damage. In much the same way, your body is slowly but surely damaged by a poor diet.

Imagine your body was a car and every single time you ate an unhealthy item a tow truck (ambulance) was required! Waiting times for ambulances would be measured in weeks and not minutes as a result.

In truth, the negative effect of poor dietary choice slowly accumulates over time. Rather than the very first exposure causing a problem, it is more the accumulative effect of thousands of individual poor dietary choices over a lifetime that may lead to the equivalent of a human tow truck having to be despatched! Therefore, take action now to limit these poor choices.

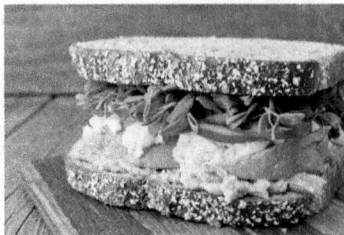

What Should We Eat?

Food pyramids give a guide as to what we should have more and less of:

More vegetables / fruit / whole grain products / nuts / olive oil / fish

Moderate amounts of red meat and dairy

Minimise packaged foods / soft drinks

Less takeaway food (especially if deep-fried or with beef patties)

On paper, it does seem easy to have a healthy diet, as all the necessary ingredients are available at any supermarket. But in this fast-paced world, time often seems short and unfortunately it is easier to take a short-cut. Quicker to miss breakfast or have a breakfast bar or drink than to sit down and have some porridge and wholemeal toast.

You need to make time — it is as simple as that.

A healthy diet is an investment in yourself — a no-brainer.

3

The Engine

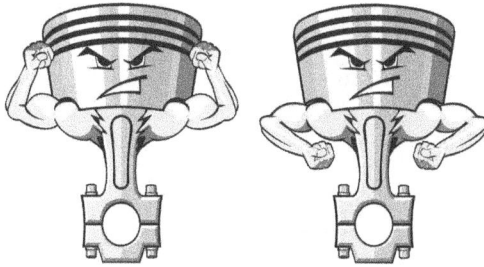

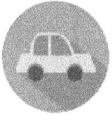

The engine is the crucial part of the car. This provides the propulsive power as well as driving — either directly or indirectly — all the other systems of the vehicle. If the motor is not working, then you are going nowhere.

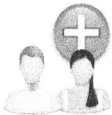

Your heart is the equivalent of the car's engine. On average it beats 70 times per minute, 4,200 times per hour, just on 100,000 times per day and well over 30

million times in a year. Each beat pumps 70 mL of blood, which equates to a volume of at least sixty Olympic swimming pools in an average lifetime!

Factors that may damage your heart:

- Blockage of the heart's own blood supply — see later re 'fuel lines'
- Raised blood pressure
- Heart valve problems
- Heart muscle damage — alcohol/other drugs/viral infection

Fuel Supply to Engine

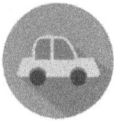

If there is a blockage in your fuel line, then the engine will be starved of fuel. The result will be that the car will run roughly at best, but most likely it will not run at all.

To prevent this requires the use of good quality fuel and replacement of the fuel filter at recommended intervals. Also, it is important that you do not let your tank run too low before filling up. This will ensure that the inevitable debris that builds up in any tank does not get drawn into the lines; a bit like the dregs in a coffee pot mucking up your nice coffee.

What about your own fuel lines?

Heart Anatomy

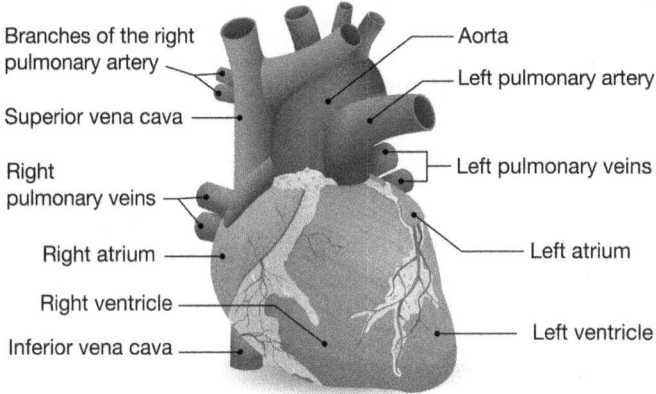

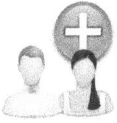

Branches of the right pulmonary artery

Superior vena cava

Right pulmonary veins

Right atrium

Right ventricle

Inferior vena cava

Aorta

Left pulmonary artery

Left pulmonary veins

Left atrium

Left ventricle

The heart pumps blood to the whole body, including itself. The heart transfers blood via two coronary arteries which run on its outer surface.

A blockage in one of these arteries can be dire... leading to a heart attack (like Nic), where there is actual heart muscle damage. This part is replaced with stiff scar tissue.

When we are young, these pipes are internally clean and therefore the blood flow is excellent. Over decades, the arteries are narrowed (called coronary heart disease) as fat deposits (atheroma) are laid down. These may, over time, cause you to have some chest discomfort when you exert yourself (i.e. angina) or cause NO trouble at all until a sudden blockage causes a heart attack.

The crucial three factors that make coronary heart disease more likely are:

- *Raised cholesterol*
- *High blood pressure*
- *Smoking*

Other important factors include:

- *Diabetes*
- *Being overweight*
- *Inactivity*
- *A family history of heart disease*

The more of these factors that you have, the more likely you will develop coronary heart disease, but again luck plays a role. Your cholesterol may be sky high but other factors are in your favor so you may never have this problem. Alternatively, you could have none of these risk factors and yet be damned unlucky.

Raised Cholesterol

Cholesterol is an essential substance found in the body and is a crucial building block of the cells. That said, an excess amount may lead to the premature buildup of atheroma (fatty deposits) in the coronary arteries, leading to their narrowing. Less blood flows as a result.

Cholesterol is made up of several types, either desirable or not — the main ones being HDL (good) and LDL (bad). The former is protective, while the latter in large amounts, particularly in those who have had previous heart attacks, is an indicator of a higher long term risk of further problems.

General targets for cholesterol mmol/l (mg/dL), approx:

Total cholesterol — 5.5 or less (200)

HDL cholesterol — 1.0 or more (40)

LDL cholesterol — 2.5 or less (100)

Treatment of raised cholesterol consists of:

Healthy eating

Loss of weight, if appropriate

Exercise

Medication

If cholesterol is deemed to be too high, especially when all other factors are considered, a statin might be prescribed. If you are diabetic or have had previous heart problems, you may be advised to take medication for a cholesterol level that an otherwise well person would not be. Your doctor will be able to calculate your risk of heart disease and therefore advise you on what is appropriate for your individual situation.

High Blood Pressure

This is common, and usually silent. Symptoms such as headaches or visual problems are rare, unless the levels are very high. For the majority with raised blood pressure (including myself), there is no obvious cause. Family history can certainly be a factor.

As well as increasing your risk of heart disease, raised blood pressure is a large factor in strokes (brain damage due to lack of blood): another very serious, life-altering medical event.

Blood pressure is expressed like a fraction, the classic text book figure being 120/80. These figures are a measure of the high and low blood pressure readings with each heartbeat. The elastic nature of the larger blood vessels allows for the flow of blood to be reasonably smooth, despite the intermittent nature of the heart's pumping action.

There is no single ideal reading but a whole range of readings which may be acceptable depending on individual circumstances. Some young women may have a reading of 90/60, which is normal for them but would not be tolerated well by others. As a general rule, consistent readings greater than 140/85 are considered to be elevated and need further attention.

Basic measures suggested to lower elevated blood pressure — before the use of medication — include the following:

- *Minimal added salt*

- *Exercise*
- *Weight control, if appropriate*

If, after several months, there has been no reasonable response to this or if the initial readings are very high, then medication will be needed to lower the blood pressure to the desirable level. Often more than one tablet may be required.

Interestingly, blood pressure does vary considerably. Readings at the clinic may be higher than they may be at home — this is known as 'white coat hypertension'. In light of this, it is often recommended to have some home readings done, either by way of a series of readings with a monitor (either bought or hired) or via a 24 hour monitor. The latter is a little cumbersome as it requires you to wear a cuff on your arm and a small monitor on your body to record the thirty or so readings. However, the information gained is important as it will clarify if you have raised blood pressure or not. Treatment can then be commenced in the full knowledge that it is required.

I often lend patients a monitor to use for a week to record twenty or so readings. They then (hopefully) return the following week with the useful information and the monitor. I have had no losses yet, although I do record their names just in case of a no-show!

Treating blood pressure can be frustrating at times. Often I detect a patient as having an elevated reading when they have attended for another reason and I have then given them some basic advice about what they may be able to do to correct it, assuming that it might always be elevated. I advise them to return in a month or so to have it rechecked. Many do not return as requested, so I have a reminder system to alert me of this. In the event of a no-show, a letter is then sent out and further follow-up encouraged. The lifetime risk of untreated blood pressure warrants this type of follow up.

Smoking

It has been known for decades that tobacco smoking is heavily linked to heart disease and many other disease states, including lung cancer and chronic lung disease. My own father requires home oxygen for this very reason. With all the remedies at hand, there is no excuse in these modern days to continue to smoke.

That said, having started to smoke it is not an easy habit to cease. It is a true addiction. Ask your doctor about the numerous ways that can be used to help you. Of course, unless you seriously wish to stop, there is no one-fix solution. Check on the internet for useful advice provided by government and other agencies as well.

4

Fluids

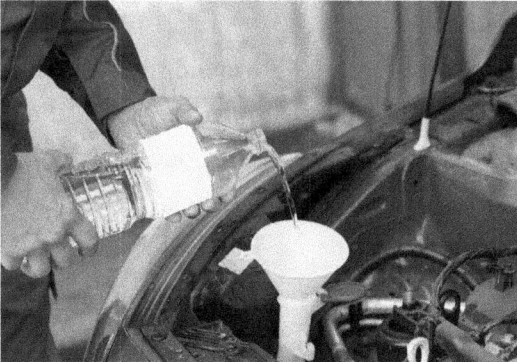

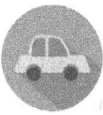

Cars have seven different types of fluids – all playing a crucial role:

- *Engine oil*
- *Coolant*
- *Transmission oil*
- *Power steering oil*
- *Brake oil*
- *Air conditioner coolant*
- *Washer fluid*

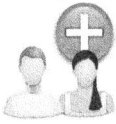

Unlike a car, you only need one fluid — fresh water! How much? Approximately 1.5-2 litres per day.

Of course, no matter what you are drinking, it is predominantly made up of water. Tea and coffee are fine in moderation, as is milk.

Dietary aspects may play a role in what you may be able to drink. Lactose intolerance may restrict the intake of cow's milk.

Generally it is strongly advised to avoid sugary drinks, including bottled fruit juices, as they simply add more dietary calories and also increase the risk of tooth decay. Even the intake of no-calorie drinks with their artificial chemical sweeteners should be minimised.

To state the obvious, it is hard to go past the simplicity of fresh water. Why spend money on products that are either harmful, provide no benefit at all, or both?

Sports drinks are of little benefit to anyone unless you are in the elite group. Alcohol in excess has multiple serious issues. These may include the risks of disinhibited behaviour, like aggression and reduced driving ability, while acutely inebriated. At the other extreme are the well-recognised complications of long term excessive intake over a lifetime. These may include: serious damage to the brain, liver and heart, just to name a few, as well as the social consequences of recurrent intoxication.

What is the safe limit of alcohol intake?

For all — no more than two (2) standard drinks on any day will reduce the lifetime risk of alcohol-related disease. Remember that a standard glass of wine is only five ounces (147 ml), so a generous home glass of wine may be closer to *two* standard drinks!

And importantly, drinking no more than four (4) standard drinks will reduce the risk of alcohol-related injury on that single occasion, e.g. accident/violence/drowning, etc.

5

Additives / Supplements

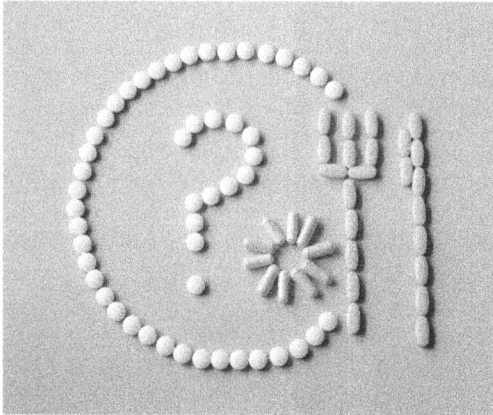

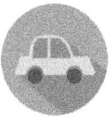

Additives for engine oil and fuel are heavily advertised as promoting engine protection, greater fuel efficiency and longer engine life. Studies reveal few that make any significant difference, and their cost is not trivial. My car's manual simply says: 'additives may adversely affect your engine or transmission performance and durability'.

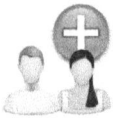

The vitamin supplement industry has become a multi-billion dollar worldwide enterprise. It is built on our wish to be as healthy as possible and the natural inclination to look for a simple fix for our problems. Spending five minutes in the vitamin aisles of a pharmacy is very interesting; watching customers reading the different labels, matching up their problems with the claimed benefits of the products on the shelf.

Some examples of the claims printed on the labels are as follows:

Multivitamin – 'support during stress / assists energy levels / stamina and vitality / based on scientific evidence'

Liver Detox – 'liver health support / helps relieve indigestion and bloating / based on scientific and traditional evidence'

Children's Fish Oil – 'to help support brain health, learning and behaviour / based on 25+ years research'

What can I say…? The claims are so vague as to be worthless, yet somehow these are allowed to be made. Unfortunately, customers who trust the printed information are being duped.

The problem is that we are gullible and tend to seek an easy answer to our current woes. We hope that by taking supplements, we will either be able to address these issues or maintain our present good health.

When going for my licence as a teenager I discovered I was short-sighted. At the time I am sure that if there had seen some drops or other treatment that claimed a remedy for poor vision

I would have most likely tried them in desperation.

Do supplements have a place? As my practice colleague Guenter advises, we all need vitamins and minerals. It is possible that we are deficient in one or another, despite a perceived reasonable diet. It is not practical to check the levels of all of these, so there is no real harm in taking a single multivitamin and mineral tablet daily to help keep these topped up. These are not that expensive.

Just do not expect to feel any better for having taken them, yet know that perhaps they may help your health in the long run. Of course they may make no difference at all — but at least no harm will have been done.

However, the main role of supplements is in proven deficiency states. If you have been tested and found to be low in iron, the first step is to work out why there is a deficiency. Is your diet low in red meat? Are you not absorbing iron properly due to coeliac disease? Are you losing blood in your bowel motions due to piles or an unknown bowel cancer? Excess menstrual loss may be the cause?

Once the cause is sorted out, then replacement of the iron can be commenced. The same applies to being low in vitamin B12 and vitamin D, etc.

In summary, by all means take a multivitamin daily, but avoid taking other products in the hope of feeling better *unless you have a proven deficiency*. Improving your overall diet should be your main aim. If you are tired or stressed, do not expect to find the answer in a bottle. Improve your diet, aim for more sleep, find time to exercise, and if you still feel tired then go to see your doctor for further advice and possible formal investigation.

6

Exterior Care / Cleanliness

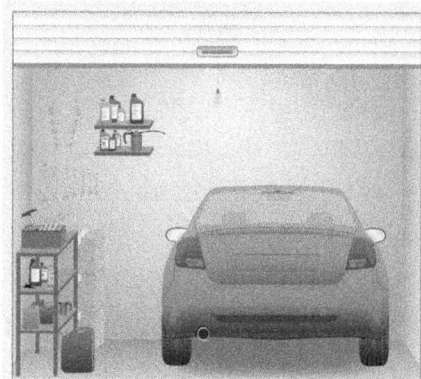

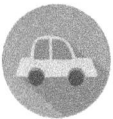

The owner's manual sets out much advice about keeping the exterior of the car in pristine condition. This includes the exterior paint work, the lights, the windows and wheel trim as well as the interior, including the seats and fittings. I doubt that this section is often read but nevertheless it is an important area.

Protecting your car's exterior from the elements, such as rain, hail and sun, is crucial in maintaining the paint work. Having your vehicle parked in a garage will make a big difference. A well protected vintage car is a pleasure to see, whether on the road or in a formal display.

Bubbles of rust poking through the car's duco are a sign of impending cosmetic disaster and need attention before they become worse and need large scale panel work.

Skin

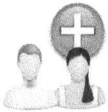

Daily showering with the use of a mild soap is important. One of the most important discoveries in the 19th century was that of Germ Theory. This proposed that individual germs could cause specific illnesses. The spread of such illnesses could be reduced dramatically by the simple act of adequate hand washing. Hence the importance of this, especially before meals and after attending the toilet. Attempts at hand washing that resemble the symbolic hand washing by a priest at a religious service are not sufficient. Take the time to do it properly. Going to the toilet at a sporting event reveals the range of people's hygiene skills — from no attempt at all to a most thorough routine.

Your exterior also needs protection. Our skin shows signs of aging over the decades. Much of this is related to the aging effects of UV radiation. For this reason, your best skin is found on your buttocks — your best as far as your skin is concerned

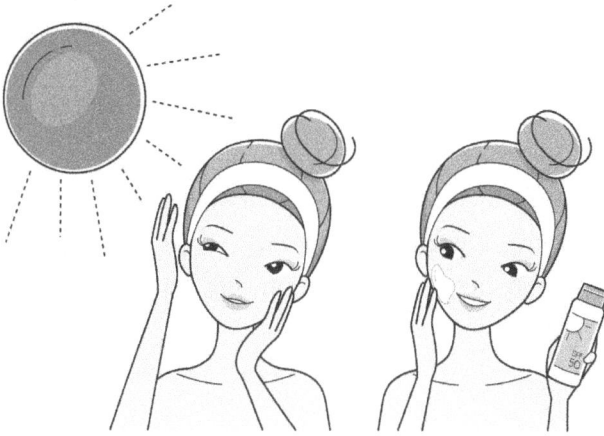

is definitely behind you! As well as making you look older, UV radiation leads to an increased risk of skin cancer, including melanoma. The risk accumulates over a lifetime — so protect your children while they are under your control, and trust that they will continue this in the long term.

High protection sun creams should be used as much as possible. These are best put on initially before you go out. You are much more likely then to put the cream on adequately if you are not rushed and have the aid of a mirror. Naturally, they may need to be reapplied after two hours or so, but at least the first application would have been well applied. Of course, covering up via a hat, sensible clothing and natural shade is also very important.

The older generations are now paying the cost of their long term sun exposure. Many elderly patients attend nowadays for treatment of solar keratoses (rough skin related to sun damage which may turn cancerous) as well as established skin cancers.

Sunburn was a known problem in years gone by, but what was not known was the long term, irreversible damage that came with it. Research suggests that one serious episode of sunburn with secondary blistering does increase your life-long risk of skin cancer. So the modern generation has no excuse for not protecting their skin.

Eyes

UV radiation is harmful and may lead to cataracts. Hence the film star routine of sun glasses does actually make sense. Being short sighted, my contact lenses provide some additional UV protection.

For those who have no known eye problems, having an eye check every 2-3 years is sufficient — more often if you are wearing glasses already. Once you hit your fifties, you may then find that you are having trouble reading and may need prescription glasses.

Appropriate eye protection is essential if you are partaking in any potentially serious activity such as whipper snipping, grinding or welding. One ounce of bad luck combined with some complacency could lead to the permanent loss of vision. I always leave my safety glasses on a specific hook in the garage and so far, they have always been there when I have needed them.

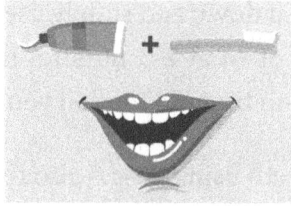

Teeth

The majority of gum and dental disease could be prevented through better attention to diet as well as better teeth cleaning routines. Recently a patient attended with the issue of bad breath. Her teeth were in poor condition, as were her gums. She was surprised when I advised her that she should clean her teeth twice daily and for 2-3 minutes on each occasion. Her previous routine was a single short brush per day. This, combined with a poor diet, had led to her current dire situation.

Time and technique is crucial for teeth cleaning. Also, a good tooth brush is important. Ensure that it is soft and looks close to brand new. Remember, you do not have to brush hard to be effective.

Even though we all like to multitask, when it comes to cleaning teeth you are best to stay anchored in front of the mirror and ensure that you clean ALL surfaces of your teeth and gums for 2-3 minutes. Walking around the house and doing something else (as I have been guilty of in the past, a habit I picked up from my father) will not do. It is hard to do the task adequately if you are not giving it your full attention. No matter how practised you are, it is unlikely to be sufficient. If you have your mobile phone with you, put it down and simply use it as a timer initially to give you a sense of what 2-3 minutes is like. Many electric brushes have a built-in timer to remind you when the time is up.

Cleaning between teeth using floss is also important, if you have the patience. Many dentists advise that you should only floss the teeth you want to keep! Both flossing and good teeth cleaning helps keep your gums healthy.

Regular dental check-ups are important. It is advised by the dental profession that these should be six-monthly. Yet cost is a huge factor that makes this impractical for many. Sadly, for the majority of the population, dental care is sought only when a problem arises as evidenced by oral pain or swelling.

Develop a routine where you perform these tasks of washing and cleaning thoroughly without having to think about them. When our kids were very young I 'tried' to do this by talking about the 'package'. This was simply the twice-daily routine of cleaning your teeth, rinsing your mouth and washing your face. They cringe now at the mere mention of the term, but they have not forgotten it either I suspect! Whether they still do it now is another matter.

All these basic hygiene matters should be as automatic as doing up your shoelaces; done so often and so well that you can do them without any thought. There simply should be no other way.

7

Tyres

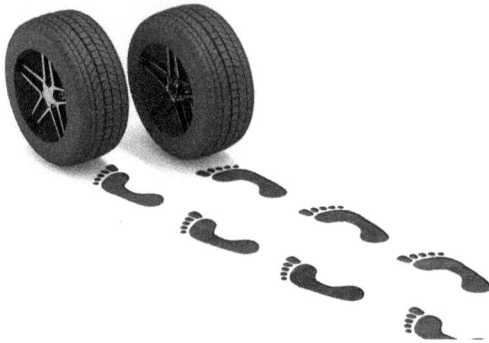

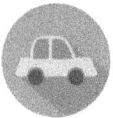

The tyres are one of the most neglected parts of a car. They are the contact point with the road. This connection must be secure for driving to be as risk free as possible. The power of the engine is driven through the tyres as is the stopping power of the brakes. Tread depth, tyre condition and inflation rates are all crucial to the performance of a car. Don't skimp when it comes to buying good quality tyres. Your life may well depend on it.

As you approach your car each morning, try to develop the habit of looking at the car tyres to ensure that they are inflated. Every month (at least) check the pressures, including the spare in the boot… even though it is a hassle! That's the time to find out that the spare is flat, not when you need it in the middle of the night at the side of the road. Luckily, Nic had made sure that his spare was well looked after.

Remember, tyre wear and car performance is heavily dependent on the tyre pressures.

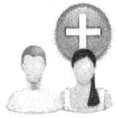

Feet also are commonly ignored until something happens. Usually pain will draw your attention to a problem. When you think about it, the feet are the load bearers of the body and over a lifetime do more than their fair share of work.

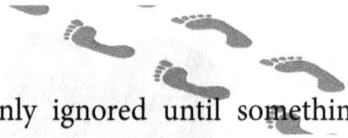

It is crucial that you make the effort to do some preventive maintenance. Ensure that your nails are trimmed short but straight. Do not cut them like your fingernails, with a curve, as this may encourage the development of an ingrown toenail. Invest in a good pair of clippers and always put them in the same place for ready use. Any persisting pain or rough areas should be investigated.

As you get older, it may be too difficult to manage your own nails for many reasons:

- Simply cannot reach them easily!
- Poor eyesight

- Inability to use the clippers well

- Thick nails, which are practically too hard to trim

You may then need to have someone else attend to them. A podiatrist may be required, especially for those with diabetes.

Foot care in the elderly is crucial. Neglect here can be the start of infection, with later amputations, particularly in those with diabetes.

8

Danger Signs

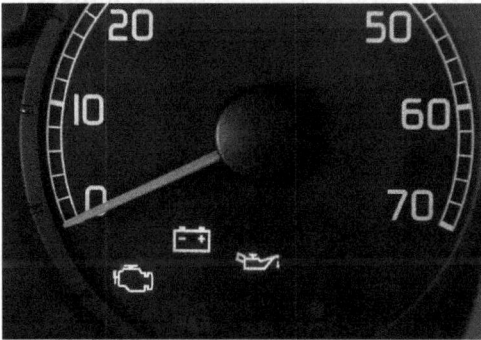

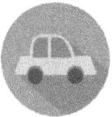

Watch the gauges:

Fuel – do not wait until the low level indicator is flashing, as some debris from the bottom of the tank may clog up the fuel line. It costs you no more to fill up the tank a little earlier.

Temperature – should be in the middle of the range once the car has warmed up. The experience of having a car that was prone to overheating when I was younger has trained me to check this very frequently.

New red light / symbol on — if a light is showing a warning, find out what it means and act accordingly. You may have to refer to the car's manual for advice! Do not simply ignore it, like my kids often do.

Lights — check occasionally that they are all operational. Shop window reflections are very useful to check these.

Check the ground where you routinely park your car — is there any sign of oil or other liquids being dropped? Note that it's common for there to be some water from the airconditioner system if it has been on.

Pay attention to the way the car sounds — is it idling and running smoothly? Brakes working well?

Every month check the level of the oil, coolant and tyre pressures.

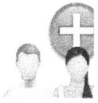

Your Danger Signs

Too many to mention them all… but some important ones are:

- Unaccustomed headaches — lasting more than a week, or sudden onset, like someone has hit you in the back of the head with a book.

- Chest pain / tightness that comes on with exercise and settles with rest

- Sudden chest pain lasting for more than five minutes in the over-forty individual, especially if NOT made worse by breathing or movement

- Shortness of breath for no apparent reason

- Feeling that your heart is going too fast

- Diarrhoea lasting longer than a week

- Blood in bowel movements — however, if less than age 30, a serious cause is less likely

- Excessive tiredness / poor appetite

- Enlarging spot on skin / non-healing sore present for more than a month

- Significant loss of weight for no obvious reason

- Prolonged sadness where you feel helpless and hopeless

- Anxiety that is affecting your personal or working life

- Recent but persisting poor sleep

- Simply do not feel right — not always easy to put into words

- Reliance on the use of excess alcohol or other drugs

- Nose bleeds — if not settling after 15 minutes, despite sitting up and squeezing the END of your nose (not the hard bit at the top!)

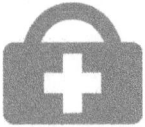

CALL an ambulance if you are suddenly very short of breath or if you have a persisting chest pain or pressure feeling for more than 10-15 minutes. Use an angina spray if prescribed one previously.

That very sudden, severe headache could have a serious cause.

Also take the time to do a first aid course or at least look up online resources and know what to do if someone collapses in front of you.

9

Driving

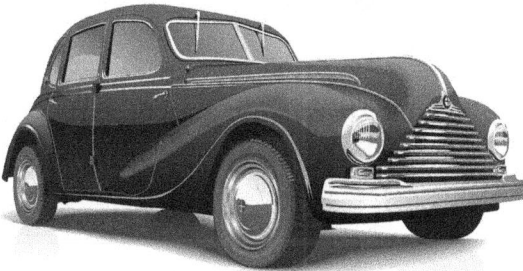

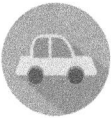

It is important that a car is used sufficiently. Short in-frequent trips do not allow the engine to warm up enough for the oil to lubricate its moving parts adequately. The end result is early wear and tear to the engine. It may take your car at least five kilometres of driving to warm up.

For this very reason, the best second-hand cars to buy are those from the country. They are most likely to have done many miles on the open road at normal running temperature, with less engine wear as a result.

An elderly patient of mine recently traded in his two-year-old car that had travelled less than two thousand kilometres. I doubt that it had ever warmed up!

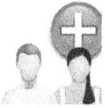

Likewise, we have to keep moving. Physical activity is crucial for your health.

According to the US Centre for Disease Control, the benefits of exercise are enormous and include the following:

- Weight control
- Reduction in risk of cardiovascular disease (heart attack and stroke)
- Reduce the risk of some cancers – colon and breast
- Reduction in risk of developing type 2 diabetes
- Bone and muscle strengthening
- Improvement in mental health
- Increased longevity
- Reduction in falls in the elderly

How much exercise?

As much as is possible! Levels of 120-150 minutes of moderate exercise per week is the ideal, but to be fair, any exercise is worthwhile. The key is to do as much as you can, given your age, health issues and other demands on your time.

What to do?

Any exercise is good — walking at a good pace, jogging, swimming, golf, tennis, cycling — just to name a few. The chance of injury is low and the benefits are enormous. You will feel better afterwards, as well as benefitting from the known positive effects long term.

You just need to keep busy, and any activity counts, including vacuuming the carpet, other housework, gardening and mowing the lawn. This is known as incidental exercise — the exercise you do without realising it! Any movement no matter how trivial it may seem is very beneficial. So think twice before you pay someone to do a household task that you could easily do. This way you can save some money and be healthier, all at the same time. Simple!

Weight training is also excellent. As well as making you look and feel better, there is marked improvement in strength and endurance. Bone density may also be improved.

Attending the local gym may be the answer. Many suburban areas these days have sporting complexes which provide a large number of exercise options. There is little excuse not to be involved.

In my area there are two council-owned gyms managed by the YMCA. The facilities are excellent: pools / spa / steam room / sauna / gym. The hours of opening are long: from 5:30 am until 10 pm daily.

My current regime (that has varied over the years) consists of 15-20 minutes in the gym doing a variety of exercises, including weight training, followed by 6-8 slow laps of the 50-metre pool. After a coldish shower to help cool down, I then head off to work. It is certainly a great way to start the day.

One word of warning — if you are middle-aged or older and have done little real activity for years, please start very slowly. If there is any doubt about your fitness, then you ought to see your doctor for a chat and a checkup first.

10

Air Intake

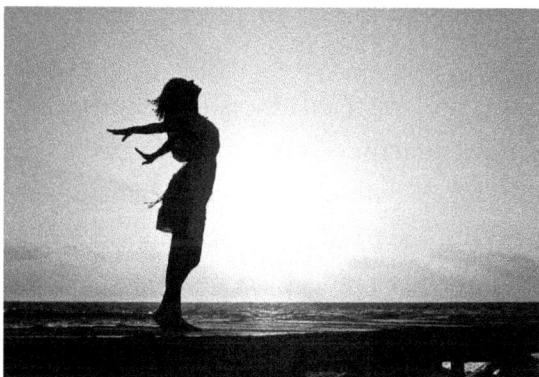

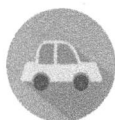

A clean air supply is crucial for the efficient running of an engine. The oxygen in the air is needed for combustion of the fuel. An air filter is essential to ensure that dust and other contaminants do not reach the inside of the engine. If they do, there will be premature wear and tear, with reduced engine power and working life. These air filters need to be replaced during regular servicing.

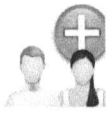

Similarly, clean air is crucial for us. Carbon monoxide and other toxic gases can be lethal. Normal air is cleaned by the hairs in the nose and by the mucus that lines the airways. Dust and other contaminants are trapped by this mucus. Small hairs known as cilia then move the mucus to the throat, where it can then be either coughed up or swallowed. The airways also humidify the air and warm it.

The mouth does not do the job as efficiently as the nose. Those who mouth breathe will often wake up with a dry mouth as a result.

Unfortunately, the upper airway is not always able to remove all potentially dangerous substances. Cigarette smoking has been clearly linked with chronic lung damage — emphysema — as well as with lung cancer. Other inhaled foreign material, such as asbestos and coal dust has shown to have similar severe problems associated with its exposure.

Do not smoke any tobacco or similar substance if you wish to live a long life. Likewise, occupational or hobby-related exposure to any type of dust requires appropriate protection, which is now readily available.

11

Cooling / Circulation System

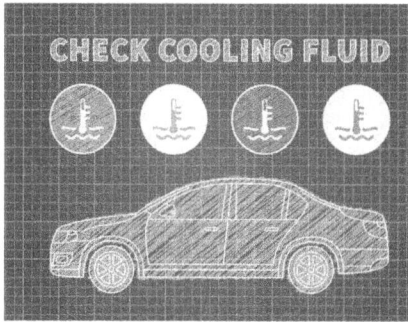

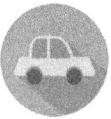

A car engine produces much heat from the combustion of fuel. This heat must be drawn away from the engine to prevent serious damage occurring. A modern car has liquid (coolant), which is circulated by the water pump around the engine to the radiator, where passing air provides the cooling effect. This liquid then flows back to the engine in a continuous fashion. The radiator cap provides for a build-up of pressure in the system, thus allowing a higher boiling point and a more efficient cooling system. Care is required; don't open this cap when the engine is still hot.

Rubber hoses connect the various components and need to be checked regularly for any obvious wear. Any weak link in this system will cause a leak of fluid and potential damage to the engine as cooling fluid is lost.

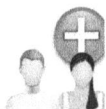

Our circulatory system consists primarily of the heart, which continuously pumps five litres of blood through a massive network of pipes (arteries and veins) to the organs of the body. This blood, having had much of its oxygen removed, is then returned to the right side of the heart, from where it is pumped into the lungs to pick up more oxygen. From the lungs it is then sent to the left side of the heart, and from there, back out to the organs. It is a continuous, never-ending circuit.

The key task of the human circulatory system is to ensure that oxygen and key nutrients are taken to all the cells of the body. As well, waste products are taken away and eliminated by the liver, lungs and kidneys. Maintenance of body temperature is in part regulated by the circulatory system.

A sudden loss of blood can have catastrophic effects. In any situation where there is damage to a major artery, with rapid blood loss, immediate action is crucial. Simple application of pressure at or above the site of bleeding either by direct pressure or via a tourniquet can be life-saving. In recent times, a surfer who had been attacked by a large shark was saved by the simple application of a tourniquet above the bite on his lower thigh. Any piece of clothing will do in such an emergency.

12

Your Mechanic

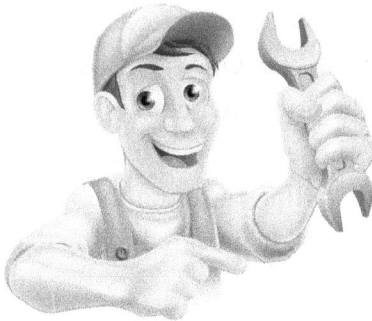

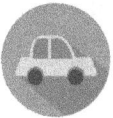

It is crucial that you have a trustworthy mechanic. Our mechanics, Dave and Pete, have been priceless over the years. It is great to be able to call upon their services at very short notice. Having had four children, with their older cars and associated problems, it has been very useful to occasionally have the broken-down car towed there overnight and be attended to the very next day. Having a relationship with a caring mechanic allows for this to occur.

Regular servicing is important. Modern cars may run for years with minimal attention as long as they have fuel and some oil. Of course if they are not serviced, problems will arise but may well be hidden for some time. The car's service manual will set out the recommended service intervals — typically 6 months / 10,000 km or 12 months / 15,000 km — whichever occurs first. A sensible owner will try to follow these guidelines if they wish to reduce the risk of preventable problems.

I have always followed these carefully, but a personal experience revealed that not everyone does. Recently I was helping one of my sons look for a used car. One car at a dealership looked great, drove nicely and the price seemed reasonable. I checked the oil and it looked old. The service book had only one visit marked in it — five years earlier! The sticker on the windscreen was so old that it was hard to read. It appeared to say that the next service was due two years ago!

Needless to say, after seeing this we headed for the hills. Sadly, I suspect many owners assume that if the car is running it must be okay. I appreciate that time can move fast yet it is important to take the time to ensure that your car is serviced regularly. It is false economy to do anything else.

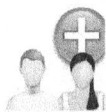

Likewise, it is important to have a doctor whom you can trust. These days there are doctors seemingly everywhere. Unfortunately, it is so easy to go to different clinics for this or that but never really belong to any. Many large medical clinics do not allow appointments to be made. Therefore, you either see the next available doctor or sit for an even longer time to see your preferred one. This is of course done for one reason alone — to have as many patients seen as quickly as possible. As a result, the quality of the service generally suffers — a scandalous result when you consider the stakes involved.

So when you really are sick and need some attention, you may not have any real rapport with any one clinic or individual doctor. It may not matter in many cases, but the truth is – it might. If you see the same doctor, then that doctor is much more likely to be thorough and sort out an ongoing problem if it is complicated. If a doctor continues to see a patient, then he or she gets to know them well. From personal experience, I find I will go the extra yard to help and be as thorough as possible.

A thorough and competent doctor will feel obliged to help you or, if unable to, be happy to refer you to a trusted specialist if required.

It is in your best interests to attend a clinic where you are not in-and-out in a flash on a routine visit. Most visits should require an unrushed history, an appropriate examination and then a reasonable explanation and a plan of action.

If you do not receive this, even if the service is free to you at the time, do not reward such poor unprofessional service with your repeat business. Your health deserves much more than this. You would not accept this poor treatment for your car, so do not take it for yourself.

Your health is much more important. Therefore, seek out someone whom you can have confidence in. If you have not had your blood pressure or weight checked in recent times, request that it be done. The truth is, you should not need to ask.

Take the time when you are there, especially if you have come for a minor problem, to request some preventive things be done. Consider whether you are up-to-date with your immunisations — if not, you could request these. Your car has items that are checked routinely and the same goes for you. If this is not happening, then go somewhere else.

Like a car, you can look good on the outside but be the complete opposite on the inside. A simple check-up, looking at your diet, activity levels, current weight and blood pressure is an excellent start.

Apart from your doctor, you may also be seeing other practitioners. I would agree that Western medicine does not have all the answers. However, be cautious when you are advised to return repeatedly for ongoing 'adjustments' to your body... as this is most unlikely to be beneficial for you. Similarly, claims to cure some ailments that seem too good to be true are probably precisely that.

13

Happiness

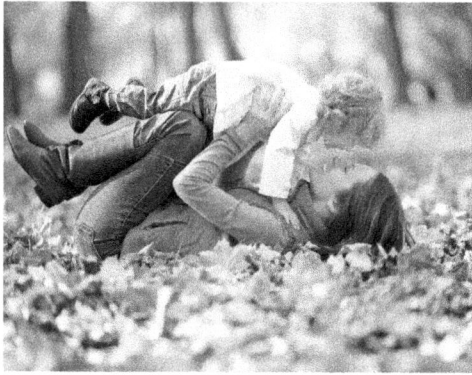

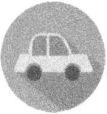

I can only assume that a car (if it had human qualities) would be most happy when it was being used and being useful. A car that sits idle all day every day would be as bored as anything. The car that was mentioned earlier — a youthful two years old and barely used — you can only imagine its frustration!

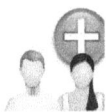

You need to be kept busy too, for your own sanity. Work provides money to live and occupies your mind and much of your time. Hobbies, family responsibilities, housework, exercise and other pastimes fill in the rest.

With boredom comes frustration. If you do not have enough to do, it's likely that you will feel dissatisfied with life and may seek some solutions for this. These may not always be beneficial for your long term health. Options such as the use of excess alcohol or other drugs may then feature.

If you are busy then you are more likely going to be happier. Even doing what may appear to be mundane tasks — like cleaning, washing and putting the bins out — are part of life and can be enjoyable in their own way. Volunteer work can be very gratifying and give much purpose. Helping those in need has its own rewards.

So make sure that you have enough to do. If you are bored — perhaps go and wash your car, or someone else's!

14

Rest

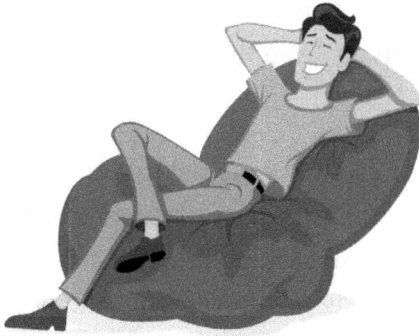

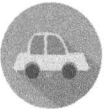

Not surprisingly, cars do not need to rest. As long as all their systems are working well and have sufficient fuel and oil, they can run nonstop until they wear out.

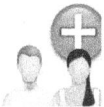

In stark contrast, humans need rest. The average person needs to have at least seven to eight hours sleep per night. Like most things in life, there is a normal range in this need for sleep. Two-thirds of the population fall within the six to nine-hour mark. In contrast, babies tend to sleep up to 16 hours per day.

Sleep deprivation has obvious consequences. You feel tired, maybe moody and your thinking will not be as sharp as usual — a huge issue if you need to be alert for your work or your driving.

The effect of tiredness is similar to having a degree of alcohol intoxication. Be wary of this effect if you are contemplating waking up early to drive long distances for a holiday. We all know the feeling when you wake up early after a late night — you feel a little foggy and need to have a shower to at least start to feel a bit better and freshen up. Even then you will not be as sharp as you should be.

Remember that sleep is as essential to your health as the air you breathe and the food you eat. Make sure that all of these are as high a quality as possible. Sleep provides a chance for your mind to rest and your body to recover from the present day and to prepare for the next.

Life should not be *all* serious. It's important to find times for leisure and enjoyment. In the 19th century, the concept of the eight hour working day came into being, with the idea that every worker had the right to eight hours of work, eight hours of recreation and eight hours of rest. This may not always be practical, but it certainly provides an ideal to aim for.

Leisure time is important to your overall wellbeing. It may be made up of a myriad of activities, including: sport, walking, cycling, swimming, various hobbies, socialising with friends and family, reading, watching TV, or attending the movies, etc.

The main message is that life should be enjoyable.

15

Safe Driving

When the car and you get together — then the fun or drama can begin.

If a car is driven well and safely, then it is a most satisfying experience. However, we have all seen situations where things have not turned out well.

The statistics on roads deaths worldwide are startling. Road deaths for 2016 were as follows:

Australia   1,200

USA   38,000

World   > 1 million

In addition, there is the hidden toll of those who have been badly hurt and their lives changed dramatically. Their numbers easily exceed the number of fatalities by many fold. I have seen several patients over the years who have had significant injuries sustained in a car accident. Years later, most are not back at work, their lives changed forever due to their injuries. For example, a young man with a compound fracture of his leg, which required multiple grafting and extended rehabilitation, is still not back at meaningful work three years post-accident.

Also, we must not forget those who have been left behind after the sudden death of a loved one. The death of a mother or father of a young family, or that of a son or daughter, creates life-changing stress.

How can you avoid being part of this? In some ways, the chance of dying or being severely injured are similar to the risk of other events in life. Some things you can control and others you cannot. Of course, you can simply be in the wrong place at the wrong time — that old random luck that plays such a role in health in general. Your task is to reduce your individual risk by changing what is within your control.

You can do this by:

- Driving within the speed limit, no matter how unreasonable certain limits appear to be.

- Taking care approaching traffic lights and glancing in the mirror to see who is behind you, in case you have to stop suddenly. There may be a car or truck right behind you who has no plans to stop!

- Keeping your distance from the car in front, i.e. a 2-3 second gap at least.

- Not changing lanes unless you have to.

- Always having a second look in each direction before you join a main road.

- Being courteous and watching out for other road users, including pedestrians.

- Looking well ahead to see what is happening beyond the car in front.

- Not driving if impaired in any way — e.g. alcohol / other drugs / sleep deprived.

First Aid

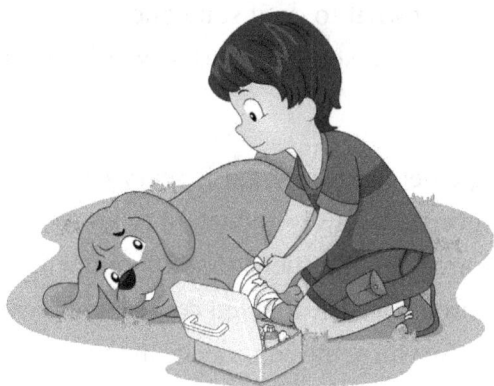

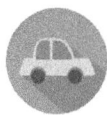

The modern car does not have many owner-serviceable parts — unless you are a real handyman. Nevertheless, you should be able to check your car's water and oil levels as well as be able to fill up your windscreen washer reservoir. Or at least have someone to do it for you.

Checking tyre pressures, including the spare, is not that difficult. Replacing faulty light bulbs can certainly be a challenge at times, often requiring marked dexterity and long fingers. The car manual may be useful in guiding you for this. Changing a tyre is not difficult once you have done it a couple of times, but some car owners do not want to get their hands dirty or are unable to get the hubcaps and nuts off to even start. Membership of the local motoring organisation can help you when things are desperate or when you need a tow. As previously stated, your own trusted mechanic is priceless.

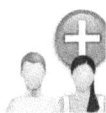

Knowing what to do if someone is critically unwell is crucial. A person collapses — would you know what to do?

Administering emergency first aid is scary even for those who are trained. Nevertheless, it is important to know. The basics are not hard — search the internet for some pointers — but more importantly, enrol in a basic first aid course. This is money well-spent and will give you some confidence in the event of an emergency. You could save a life.

Summary

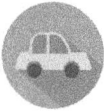

Unless you've been unlucky and bought a lemon, not maintained your car as advised, or simply driven poorly — you have every chance of having a working car that will serve you well for many years into the future. With such a vehicle, you will be able to decide if and when to change it, rather than having to urgently find a replacement when it 'unexpectedly' dies on you due to neglect.

Likewise — for your own body. Barring awful bad luck or poor decision-making throughout your life, you too have every chance of making a good age, with hopefully a vintage body too.

This is definitely in your hands. What's required is for you to continue to do these simple preventive things repeatedly, until they become automatic and part of your daily routine... healthy habits for the rest of your life.

Of course, this is the hard part, but the long-term benefits are enormous for both you and your family! So make the effort and start today.

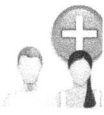

Whatever happened to Nic?

Back to Nic, the man with chest pain, who I met that Sunday afternoon.

He returned to see me ten days later, armed with a bottle of champagne to acknowledge our great effort. It was much appreciated. A great result for all — Nic survived his heart attack and has remained well since. And that was over 15 years ago.

I still see Nic when he comes in for his six-monthly checks. He is now in his early nineties, yet the memory of that day and night never fades. Good, funny memories never do.

Both he and his car are still both doing well!

Appendix

Periodic Maintenance Schedule

Every car comes with a manual that lists all the crucial maintenance tasks that need to be undertaken on a regular basis. "The periodic maintenance schedule is designed to help you receive proper performance, durability and reliability from your vehicle". It serves as a formal record of the servicing history of the vehicle and is priceless if you ever wish to sell the vehicle.

You are a brave person if you buy a used vehicle that has no service books to vouch for its service history.

If you were a car, your maintenance schedule might look a bit like this.

Individual Maintenance Schedule — minimum

Daily

These daily maintenance items are the key factors in ensuring that you remain as healthy as possible. They all seem rather mundane when listed, but they are all crucial activities that are easily done.

When done on a regular basis, they soon become habits — excellent habits that will go a long way to making you a healthier and happier person.

Wash face	Twice daily
Clean teeth	Twice daily / 2-3 minutes / soft brush — replace if frayed
Wash hands	As needed — pre meals / after toilet — use adequate technique
Diet	Ensure healthy intake / minimal processed food
Fluids	Mainly water - tap is fine - 1.5-2 litres daily
Washing	Shower - 3-5 minutes. Be mindful of the cost of a 30 minute shower!
Exercise	Walk / run / swim / house or garden work / gym workout / weights 20–30 mins daily 4–5 times per week Do what you can depending on your own limitations
Rest	Allow some downtime to relax — TV / read / meditate
Sleep	7 – 9 hours sleep regularly — take care if less / beware fatigue
Social	Interact with people — at work / home / socially
Goals	Have a plan for the day

REGULAR RITUALS

2 – 4 weekly	Trim finger and toe nails
1 – 3 monthly	Hairdresser (if you have hair!)
6 - 12 monthly	Dental check

12 monthly	
Medical check-up	Local family doctor — ideally same person, for continuity. May be more often if having ongoing issues
Goals	Have a plan for the day / month / year / your life

WARRANT OF FITNESS CHECKS – YOU

2019

Medical Practitioner - *passed*

2020

Medical Practitioner - *passed*

2021

Medical Practitioner - *passed*

2022

Medical Practitioner - *passed*

2023

Medical Practitioner - *passed*

Useful Sites

Victorian Government Better Health Channel
https://www.betterhealth.vic.gov.au

NSW Government Health sites:
https://www.health.qld.gov.au/public-health
http://www.health.nsw.gov.au/healthyliving

BMI calculator – **http://bit.ly/BMI-calc-hf**

Waist measurement – **http://bit.ly/waistmeasure**

Diseases and conditions, US Center for Disease Control and Prevention – **http://bit.ly/disease-control**

Smoking cessation advice – **http://www.quitnow.gov.au**

Children's weights, Better Health Vic – **http://bit.ly/bmi-kids**

First aid advice, St Johns – **http://bit.ly/first-aid-advice**

Healthy diet pyramid, Nutrition Aust. – **http://bit.ly/hl-pyramid**

Healthy eating guidelines, UK. **http://bit.ly/uk-healthy-eating**

The Last Word

Roger Smith (the Simple Doctor) has been a family doctor since the mid-1980s. He works in a large group practice which has provided a quality service to the community since 1978. As well as seeing patients in the clinic, the doctors attend the elderly in their own homes and in local aged care facilities — a total service.

General practice has changed immensely over the years but the basics have not. Taking a proper history, performing an appropriate examination and explaining to the patient the issues in question remain crucial. The basics of a good diet, exercise, and good routines cannot be stressed enough.

Luck plays a role, but why not make your own luck? This book explains your role in your own health. The Simple Doctor wishes you to do what you can to make your life journey as healthy as possible.

☙

DRIVE YOURSELF TO A HEATHIER LIFE